DIABETES

USING NATURAL FOODS TO MANAGE AND

CURE TYPE 1 & TYPE 2 DIABETES

MARY GRIFFIN

ISBN-13: 978-1540638229

ISBN-10: 1540638227

Why I Wrote This Book

I was compelled to write this book, *Diabetes: Using Natural Foods to Manage and Cure Type 1 & Type 2 Diabetes,* when I became aware that diabetes is a silent, insidious disease that is adversely affecting and killing a lot of people unnecessarily. Even more troubling - many people are suffering from diabetes and don't know it.

Two years ago I lost an uncle to kidney complications in what I later learned was caused by diabetes. For one and a half years of hospital visits, treatment and pain, the disease slowly ravished him and eventually led to his early death; he was not even 50 years old! The extreme financial burden to the family and the emotional pain to the wife (my aunt) and my four young cousins was unbearable. My aunt turned into a shell of an emaciated wife, struggling and praying by her husband's bedside as he struggled and slowly died from the complications of diabetes.

Beyond the pain of losing my uncle, of more concern for me is the fact that the disease is attacking children, and this is supported by the thousands of cases recorded. Children are eating unhealthy foods, leading poor lifestyles, and are less active than they should be. If the trend continues unabated we will have a sick generation where the majority of people are struggling with diabetes. Imagine the profound financial costs at the local and national level as well as the loss of life and the households this will affect.

Did you know that diabetes is now the cause of more deaths and health complications than any of the major diseases? In fact, diabetes is the modern day health crisis, killing more people than other major medical problems like cancer and AIDS.

I have made inquiries and researched diabetes extensively and feel I should share what I have learned. Further, I have included insights and information on the causes of diabetes, the risk factors which may make you vulnerable to the disease, how to prevent and shield yourself from developing the disease, and even the complications and challenges resulting from diabetes.

I sincerely hope this book plays a part in creating needed awareness and shares the lifestyle and eating habits needed to prevent and reverse diabetes.

Why You Should Read This Book

If you want to know, understand, prevent, and learn how to reverse diabetes if you already have the condition, then you should read this book. *Diabetes: Using Natural Foods to Manage and Cure Type 1 & Type 2 Diabetes* will teach you how diabetes develops and what triggers its development. Did you know that there are more than one type or form of diabetes? This book explains how each is caused.

Do you have concerns about the adverse side effects of medications that "allegedly" cure or treat diabetes? If you are overwhelmed by the sweating, the fatigue and many other harmful side effects of diabetic medications, it's time you tried the most natural and effective remedy for the management and cure of diabetes and its complications - natural foods. Organic food, if well prepared and eaten in moderation, is far better than expensive pharmaceutical drugs.

Stop giving your hard earned money to hospitals and the pharmaceutical industry to treat diabetes. Instead, save your money and learn how to lead a better lifestyle with meals that will boost your immunity and will help you end diabetes. Read *Diabetes: Using Natural Foods to Manage and Cure Type 1 & Type 2 Diabetes.*

Are you ready? Let's begin.

TABLE OF CONTENTS

CHAPTER 1

WHAT IS DIABETES?

Diabetes is a chronic metabolic disease caused by hormonal imbalance as a result of the body's inability to produce sufficient insulin for the optimal regulation and conversion of glucose leading to elevated sugar levels in the blood. Basically, a person who suffers from diabetes has too much glucose in the blood for the body to use. When diabetics eat carbohydrates or starch, which is the source of glucose, it cannot be converted or burned into energy, and instead lingers in the blood resulting in high levels of blood sugar. Excess sugar can lead to weight gain.

The pancreas is the organ responsible for the production of insulin, which is responsible for regulating how much glucose makes it into the blood stream. Glucose is the body's natural sugar produced from the breaking down and synthesis of carbohydrates.

WHO CAN GET DIABETES?

Diabetes can affect anyone at any stage of life - as a child, as a young or older adult. Within the past 15 years there has been a profound rise of people suffering or being diagnosed with diabetes and experts estimate that by the year 2030 the number will be double what it is today. The point is, diabetes is a cause for concern and it is something we should watch out for and learn how to deal with.

In fact, diabetes is leading to more deaths than cancer and AIDs and brings along with it associated illnesses and conditions such as kidney failure, amputations, heart attacks and strokes, blindness, and debilitating medical problems. Apart from the human and related costs, there are the high financial and emotional costs accruing. Diabetes takes a toll on the patient as well as those close to them.

There is good news. With the proper knowledge and care, diabetes is manageable and it is possible to cure and prevent symptoms arising as well as the resultant afflictions and complications such as heart attacks, blindness, festering wounds, amputations and the like.

TYPES OF DIABETES

There are two main types of diabetes, Type 1 and Type 2, but there are other forms of the disease such as gestational diabetes which affects women during pregnancy.

TYPE 1 DIABETES

Type 1 diabetes is a result of an immune system attack on the pancreas, known as autoimmune disease, where the insulin producing cells of the pancreas are mistaken as foreign and are destroyed. The pancreas cells, or islets, that are destroyed are the ones responsible for sensing glucose levels in the blood and are programmed to release sufficient insulin to regulate or balance blood sugar content.

With lack of insulin, sugar deposited in the blood from the digested carbohydrates and starch accumulates in the blood and the body cells are starved of energy which would have been converted by the missing insulin. This sugar that builds up in the blood stream ends up destroying the eyes, the heart, kidneys, and the nerves apart from causing other complications.

Type 1 diabetes is the more severe form of diabetes. It is also known as insulin-dependent diabetes and is sometimes referred to as juvenile diabetes because it mostly affects children even though it can develop at any stage.

Type 2 DIABETES

Type 2 diabetes is also referred to as adult onset or non-insulin dependent diabetes because it typically occurs after the age of 35, but there are recent studies showing that a growing number of younger people are suffering from this diabetes. This type of diabetes occurs when the insulin produced in the body is deficient or if the insulin released does not work properly - which is called being insulin resistant.

Type 2 diabetes is increasing rapidly with many people suffering silently as they are yet to be diagnosed. This type of diabetes is also becoming more prevalent due to poor diet and lack of exercise. Therefore, it should not be surprising that most cases are among overweight people and those that do not engage in frequent physical exercise. Genetic predisposition is also a factor in the increased occurrence of Type 2 diabetes. Some people from different races or ethnicities are more vulnerable to suffer from diabetes than others.

GESTATIONAL DIABETES

Gestational diabetes affects pregnant women and will usually disappear after giving birth; it is a pregnancy period form of diabetes. However, once someone has had gestational diabetes, they are at a higher risk of developing Type 1 or Type 2 diabetes. There is a link between the occurrence of gestational diabetes and the development of Type 2 diabetes. Many women that experienced gestational diabetes went on to develop Type 2 diabetes.

PRE-DIABETES

Pre-diabetes is a condition where blood sugar (glucose) levels are more elevated than normal, but not enough to qualify as a case of diabetes and is usually a precursor to diabetes. Many people are being diagnosed with pre-diabetes which makes the situation worrying - this is a pool of potential full blown diabetes sufferers.

SECONDARY DIABETES

Secondary diabetes is a condition of elevated blood sugar levels caused by another medical condition. It can develop as a result of pancreatic damage through a disease like chronic pancreatitis - an inflammation of the pancreas by toxins like excessive alcohol, or removal of the pancreas through surgery.

Diabetes from hormonal instability

Diabetes can be triggered by other hormonal disturbances other than insulin. These include:

- Acromegaly- Excessive growth hormone production as a result of pituitary gland tumour leading to hyperglycemia (high blood sugar).

- Cushing's syndrome- Adrenal glands produce excess Cortisol which encourages glucose elevation in the blood.

Having looked at the types of diabetes and what diabetes is, let's delve into the causes and symptoms that may indicate that you or someone you know is suffering from diabetes.

CHAPTER 2

CAUSES AND SYPMTONS OF DIABETES

How can you tell that you or someone you know may be suffering from diabetes?

Many people have diabetes (more so Type 2) but are unaware, especially when the disease is in the early stages because they do not know the signs to look out for. The symptoms listed below can point you to the fact that you or someone you know could have or be developing the disease. However, the only definite way of knowing if you have diabetes is by having your blood sugar levels evaluated by a physician.

Type 1 diabetes symptoms can manifest suddenly and are more likely than not to be life threatening. For this reason, its diagnosis is usually very fast and rather straight forward. On the other hand, Type 2 diabetes does not show any noticeable symptoms early on in many cases. It is more insidious and by the time the symptoms are noticed complications may already be present.

DIABETES SYMPTOMS

The common symptoms of Type 1 and Type 2diabetes include:

Excessive Urinating

The average person urinates 4 to 7 times a day but for the diabetic the frequency is more and this can lead to dehydration if one is not careful.

Whereas with non-diabetics, the cells are able to absorb and metabolize the glucose produced, in the diabetic the saturation of glucose in the blood causes the body to find a way to dispose of it - usually through the urine.

Dry mouth and persistent thirst

As a result of dehydration brought about by loss of water through urine, your body will demand more fluids making you feel thirsty and leaving your mouth less moist and dry.

Itchy skin and skin infections

With almost all the fluids in your body being converted to urine, your skin will may suffer from dryness leading to itchiness and even infections.

Blurred vision and blindness

Diabetes can cause poor vision and eventually blindness due to destruction of micro-vessels in the eyes. The lenses swell, lose their shape and eventually cannot focus.

Yeast infections

Yeast infections are quite common in diabetics with the fungal growth appearing in moist warm areas or folds such as the groin, between the toes and fingers, and under the breasts for women.

Since yeast feeds off sugar, and with the excess glucose in the body, coupled with moist areas the yeast has fertile ground to grow.

Festering wounds

If you notice that sores on your skin or cuts are taking longer than usual to heal, you may want to check if you have diabetes. Festering and slow healing wounds may be due to nerve damage caused by high blood sugar.

Tingling feeling or numbness in hands or feet

This is another consequence of nerve damage as a result of high blood sugar. You will feel numbness or a tingling sensation in the extremities and sometimes even pain.

Weight loss; Type 1 diabetes

Since the glucose is not being converted to energy your body will burn body fat and muscle tissue to get the energy your body requires. Usually, weight loss in diabetics is not planned; your eating habits have not changed but you still lose weight.

Fatigue

Usually, as a result of the changes that are happening in the body, you are likely to feel tired most of the time. The weight loss and muscle atrophy from the body's attempt to compensate leads to fatigue.

Nausea and vomiting

In some serious Type 1 diabetes cases, nausea and vomiting is experienced as a result of the body burning fats to produce energy. In this process, chemicals called ketones are produced and can sometimes accumulate in the blood at dangerously high levels leading to a condition called ketoacidosis which is life threatening. The ketones lead to nausea and vomiting.

Type 2 diabetes symptoms:

- Feeling hungry more than usual
- Weight gain
- Irritability and mood swings
- Headaches and dizziness
- Cramping of the leg

HOW TO FIND OUT IF YOU HAVE DIABETES

If you are showing any of the signs noted above, you should visit a doctor and complete a proper medical evaluation to confirm if you have diabetes. The doctor will usually order a fasting blood glucose test - you will be required to fast for 8 hours before your blood sample is taken and tested for sugar levels. The normal glucose levels for a non-diabetic is between 70-110 mg/dl, so if your reading is higher than 140 you may be diabetic.

WHAT ARE THE CAUSES OF DIABETES?

Diabetes, in most cases, is caused by a combination of issues. There are certain things that make it easier for you to develop diabetes. You may not get diabetes directly from these things but they increase the chances of you being diabetic.

As you have already learned, Type 1 diabetes is principally caused by problems and damages from insufficient insulin production; however, Type 2 diabetes is primarily caused by unhealthy lifestyle and eating habits.

Metabolic syndrome

Metabolic syndrome refers to a cluster of conditions that are generally present in people with insulin resistance and includes the following: high blood pressure, excess midriff weight, high blood sugar levels, high cholesterol readings and elevated triglycerides.

Obesity or excess body weight

Obesity and excess body weight is a modern day problem caused by sedentary lifestyles and unhealthy eating habits. This is also a big contributor to the growing number of diabetes cases.

Excess weight can cause insulin resistance, especially in those with a lot of weight around the stomach or waist. This is why many children today are developing Type 2 diabetes.

Poor body molecular cells communication

If the cells in your body do not communicate properly and the production of insulin and regulation of glucose is distorted it can lead to diabetes.

If the cells that make insulin send out the wrong amount of insulin at the wrong time, your blood sugar get thrown off. High blood glucose can damage these cells, too.

Unhealthy daily habits and lifestyle

- Lack of or little physical exercise
- Smoking
- Stress
- Sleeping problems (either too little or too much)

RISK FACTORS FOR DIABETES

Listed below are the characteristics that increase the likelihood of you developing diabetes. The risk factors for Type 1 diabetes are not very well known or understood as much as those for Type 2 diabetes.

- Family history of diabetes, especially Type1
- Diseases and infections of the pancreas
- Obesity or excess weight
- High blood pressure
- High triglycerides and cholesterol
- Inactive lifestyle
- Mid to old age
- Polycystic ovary syndrome
- Insulin resistance

HOW TO PREVENT DIABETES

There are some simple things that can be done right now to help prevent the development or reduce the effects of diabetes.

Lose weight

As you know by now, excess weight puts you at risk of developing diabetes. If you are obese, get on a weight loss plan by dropping 10% of the excess weight you carry. Losing weight can cut the likelihood of Type 2 diabetes by half.

Exercise - Be active

Physical exercise and activity is important in weight management and keeping diabetes at bay. Engage in a form of physical exercise or activity for at least 30 minutes per day. Exercise burns glucose and helps in its regulation.

Eat healthy

A healthy diet is by far the most important component to manage and prevent diabetes.

Stay away from daily or regular intake of highly processed carbohydrates, sweets and fizzy drinks and saturated fats. These foods and beverages should not be part of your regular diet at all. You should also limit the amount of processed and red meat you eat.

Later in this book you will learn the healthy natural foods you need to eat to safely manage and cure diabetes symptoms and complications.

Quit smoking

Nicotine is not good for you whether you are diabetic or not. The damage caused by nicotine to the body can lead to the development of diabetes or trigger more complications for one who is already diabetic.

CHAPTER 3

CHALLENGES CAUSED BY DIABETES

Diabetes can cause lots of challenges and severe complications. It is important to be aware of these potential problems and prepare a plan to prevent them or how to deal with them if they appear.

Diabetes can cause challenges such as eye problems to more severe problems that require amputation of lower limbs. This chapter will highlight some of the major problems that are faced by those with diabetes and how to deal with them.

FOOT PROBLEMS

Foot problems are very common among those suffering from diabetes. Even ordinary problems like athlete's foot or a small cut can develop into bigger problems. In fact, foot problems are probably the main area of concern for many people who have diabetes.

Foot problems usually develop due to nerve damage in the foot area, leading to loss of sensation, tingling or a burning or stinging pain. If the loss of sensation occurs it can lead to one hurting or injuring a foot and not realising it.

The following are the more severe foot problems:

Changes on the skin

Dehydration can cause the skin on your foot to become dry leading to cracking and peeling. This condition is caused by dead nerves in the foot responsible for the regulation and release of oils and moisture in that area. If you are diabetic, make sure that your skin is well oiled and moisturised to prevent any damage and do not oil between the toes as the extra moisture can lead to infection.

Callus and corns

Hardening of the skin on the feet occurs much faster in diabetics. If calluses or corns are not trimmed this can lead to foot ulcers and wounds. Get a pumice stone to scrub down the developing corns and calluses and oil your foot after every bath or shower.

Ulcers

Foot ulcers mostly occur on the heel or under the big toe usually as a result of ill-fitting shoes. If these ulcers are neglected it can become infected and lead to the amputation of a limb.

Poor blood circulation

Due to the atrophy of blood vessels and nerves in the foot the ability to fend off infection and heal is compromised. The hardening and narrowing of these blood vessels can be further aggravated by habits like smoking which can harden the arteries.

Do not smoke and avoid foods with high cholesterol. Exercise and massages are also good to improve blood circulation.

Amputation

Because of reduced blood circulation in the foot, diabetics have a higher likelihood of getting a leg amputated than any other group of people. Foot ulcers and leg infections that will not heal is the reason for the high incidences, which is due to nerve disease and atrophy and reduced blood circulation in feet.

Amputations are entirely preventable. All you need is to give your feet proper care and attention. Regularly check your feet and get the appropriate footwear to prevent injury or scarring.

Neuropathy

Neuropathy refers to nerve atrophy and this leaves the diabetic with reduced pain sensation to feel a foot injury.

DIABETIC KETAOCIDOSIS AND KETONES

Diabetic ketoacidosis is a condition where, caused by inadequate insulin the cells are unable to get sufficient sugar needed for energy production; the body resorts to burning fats for energy producing ketones. Ketones are chemical by products created from breaking down fat. A build-up of ketones in the body leads to elevated acidity called ketoacidosis, which is a very serious condition as it poisons the blood and can lead to death.

NEPHROPAHTY OR KIDNEY DISEASE

Diabetes can lead to kidney failure, a condition where the kidneys lose the ability to remove waste from the blood and balance fluids.

When protein is digested, waste products are created and it is the kidney that clears the blood and the body of these wastes. When there is a high-level of blood sugar the kidneys can become overworked trying to filter the blood.

Eventually, the stress on the kidneys causes them to lose their filtering ability and the waste products build up in the blood. Once the kidneys fail the patient will need dialysis or a kidney transplant in order to stay alive.

HYPERTENSION OR HIGH BLOOD PRESSURE

Blood pressure is the force of blood flow in the blood vessels. When blood moves through your blood vessels with a lot of pressure, it is known as high blood pressure or hypertension. The heart works much harder when blood pressure is high and the chances of suffering heart complications and diabetes increases.

STROKE

A stroke is the sudden interruption of blood flow to part of the brain, leading to brain tissue damage in the affected area. It is caused when a blood clot blocks a blood vessel in the brain or neck cutting of supply of blood to the brain.

If you have diabetes, your chances of having a stroke are one and a half times higher than someone that does not have diabetes. It is imperative that you take steps to lead a healthy life in order to lower the risks of having a stroke. Keep your blood sugar, blood pressure and cholesterol in check by eating a healthy diet, getting physical exercise, and not smoking.

HYPEROSMOLOR HYPERGLYCEMIC NONKETOTIC SYNDRONE (HHNS)

HHNS is a serious diabetic condition prevalent in older persons and affects those with Type 1 or Type 2 diabetes that is not well managed or treated and is caused by another infection or illness.

Once blood sugar levels become elevated the body tries to rid itself of the excess sugar through urine. As the frequency of urination declines and the color darkens, the diabetic will experience acute thirst and dehydration. If the condition persists, the acute dehydration can lead to seizures, a coma, or even death.

GASTROPARESIS

Gastroparesis is a disorder that affects those with Type 1 or Type 2 diabetes and causes the stomach to take longer than normal to expel its contents. The vagus nerve, which controls the movement of food through the digestive tract, if damaged or stops working, movement of food will be slowed or halted. Gastroparesis can aggravate diabetes by making it difficult for the body to manage blood glucose.

Summary

This chapter identified some of the major challenges and complications that a diabetic may face as he or she deals with the disease. By knowing the obstacles that can be in your way to recovery, you have a step on the disease. Work towards eliminating these problems if you are dealing with any or work to prevent the onset of these problem by following the advice in this book.

You should read and find out more about these issues and how to deal with them. There is so much material that could further help bolster your knowledge and fight against diabetes. Apart from talking with your doctor and reading additional material about diabetes, speak with those living with the condition or those that are cured and learn from their experiences. Sharing experiences is a great way of getting more insights that will help you overcome diabetes for a healthier and happier life.

CHAPTER 4

NATURAL FOODS TO MANAGE AND CURE DIABETES

In this chapter you will learn the proper foods to include in your diet to effectively manage and cure symptoms and complications that arise as a result of diabetes. Diabetes, a metabolic disease that affects other bodily functions, parts and systems in the body, requires that you eat healthy foods that have the ability to not only manage the condition but cure and leave you healthy and well.

Diabetes is undoubtedly on the rise, but it is possible to prevent a lot of these cases, and even reverse some, if only the right foods are eaten. Preventing and curing diabetes complications does not mean eating bland or poor tasting food. On the contrary, it is eating tasty - well balanced food to boost your energy and improve your mood. Eating more fresh fruits and vegetables, less refined carbohydrates, good fats and lean protein to boost blood-sugar balance, you dramatically decrease your chances of getting diabetes and can reverse any symptoms you may have.

Since diabetes is a blood sugar concentration disease, you clearly do not want to eat foods that will bring about elevated glucose levels in the blood. Eat natural foods that are rich in nutrients that will fight diabetes and the complications thereof, as well as strengthen your immune system to fend off any other problems that could lead to diabetes.

NATURAL FOODS YOU SHOULD EAT

The following are some of the best foods to include in your diet to help you manage and cure diabetes and the resultant symptoms:

Green leafy vegetables

These are the best vegetables to help you fight diabetes for reversal and prevention. By eating more green vegetables, you lower the risk of developing Type 2 diabetes. A daily serving of green veggies lowers the risk by 9%. Eat more spinach, kales and benefit from the lutein and carotenoid properties to help with vision and prevent debilitating eye problems. Eating green leafy vegetables will also give you fibre, iron, vitamins B and vitamin C.

Citrus fruits

It has been found that diabetics have low levels of vitamin C. Eat more lemons, oranges and the like to empower your body to fend off the complications that may be lurking. Citrus is great for boosting immunity, are low in fat content and are rich in fibre.

Apples

Apples have healthy natural sugar, low levels of calories and high fibre which will fill you up and keep you from over eating. They also contain antioxidants which are natural disease fighting constituents. Include an apple in your breakfast or eat one in between meals as a snack.

Avocado

For the benefit of monounsaturated fat, avocado is one of the best fruits available. Avocado is slow to digest and helps in the regulation of blood sugar by inhibiting elevations of sugar in the blood. As a source of good healthy and natural fats, it can help in the reversal of insulin resistance leaving you with well-balanced and regulated sugar levels. Use avocado in a sandwich in place of your usual spreads like margarine or butter.

Barley

Barley is a very healthy substitute for white rice and is even better than brown rice.

Studies have shown that barley can reduce and steady blood sugar after consumption. Barley has fibre and other chemical constituents that act to slow digestion and absorption of carbohydrates, which as you know is converted to sugar. Barley can be used as an ingredient in soups or as a side dish in a meal.

Beans

It is recommended that diabetics eat beans at least twice a week. Beans contain a soluble fibre that is able to subdue a spike in blood sugar. And because of the protein nutrients, beans are a good replacement for meats; especially red meat which, if not lean, is not suitable for diabetes management and treatment. Include beans, chicken peas, and kidney beans in your diet for maximum diabetes fighting benefits.

Lean beef

If you have to eat red meat go for lean beef. Just like most proteins, it is slow to digest and keeps you full longer, thus avoiding the temptation of unhealthy snacks as well as helping in the regulation of blood sugar levels.

Berries

Blueberries have a compound called anthocyanin which is thought to help fight diabetes by lowering blood sugar through the stimulation of insulin production.

Broccoli

Remember how much broccoli was a problem to eat as a child? Well, it turns out broccoli is great for those who are dealing with diabetes. Apart from the fibre, it has antioxidants and vitamin C as well as chromium minerals. Chromium is known for the ability to control sugar levels in the blood for long periods of time. Include broccoli in your diet.

Carrots

Despite the murmurs about carrots raising blood sugar. Carrots do not have a negative effect for people who are dealing with blood sugar problems. The sugar levels in carrots are low. Beta-carotene, which carrots contain plenty of, has been linked to healthier blood sugar regulation and a lower risk of diabetes.

Non-starch vegetables

These are the non-green vegetables like onions, mushrooms, garlic, etc. They are the best for blood sugar as they have very minimal effect if at all. They are rich in fiber and phytochemicals.

Fish

One of the riskiest complications that accompany diabetes is heart disease. If one eats fish once a week the risk of heart diseases decreases significantly. The omega 3 fatty acids in fish reduce inflammation in the body which contributes to heart disease and insulin resistance among other ailments.

Seeds and nuts

Seeds and nuts are rich in healthy good fats, protein and fibre. They are also rich in magnesium which plays a key role in the absorption of insulin by body cells. Include seeds and nuts like flaxseed, sunflower, sesame, pumpkin, peanuts, and cashew nuts in your diet.

Since seeds and nuts have high fibre and protein content, they are digested slowly thus reducing their conversion to sugar and making them great for blood sugar regulation.

Yogurt and milk

Yogurt and milk have protein and calcium nutrients which helps towards weight loss. And as you know, excess weight and obesity can contribute to development of diabetes and further. These nutrients also fight insulin resistance.

Olive oil

Olive oil is the healthiest edible oil around and has strong anti-inflammatory properties that fight diabetes and heart disease, and unlike some oils does not enhance insulin resistance. Olive oil also reduces the digestion process so that the possibility of elevation of blood sugar is reduced.

Whole-grain bread

To effectively cure and manage diabetes you should avoid eating refined and processed foods, which when broken down is converted to sugar in your body. Eating refined flour and processed food is like eating sugar. The result is an elevation of sugar levels in the blood. To beat diabetes, stick to eating whole grain bread. Whole bread slows digestion and regulates the amount of sugar released in the blood.

Sweet potatoes

Sweet potatoes have properties that fight diseases, slow digestion, and help lower cholesterol levels. They also have carotenoids - the chemical responsible for the colours (reddish or yellowish) in the sweet potatoes, and are helpful in the absorption of insulin as well as chlorogenic, which lowers insulin resistance.

DIABETES FIGHTING MEAL PLANS

Apart from eating the healthy natural foods that will help in the regulation and balance of blood sugar in your body, it is more critical that you get on a balanced diet for overall health benefits and nutrition. Remember, diabetes brings along with it other problems and complications and is sometimes triggered by other illnesses and health problems. A meal plan arrived at together with your doctor's input (who actually knows something about nutrition; many don't) will help you in your fight to beat diabetes more efficiently.

A diabetes fighting meal plan is a designed set of meals or set of nutrients and eating habits that are deliberately chosen for the effective management of diabetes and cure of symptoms or complications. The plans are designed to conform to your schedule to ensure that you get the requisite nutrients for your body.

This approach to management and treatment of diabetes problems is insightful and necessary as not everyone can accommodate the same meal plan. Everyone has to create a meal plan that works for them. A sound meal plan involves controlling the food portions you consume and monitoring the carbohydrates intake. The following are some methods you may consider:

Monitoring carbohydrates intake

This method of meal planning involves counting and controlling how much carbohydrates you consume per meal.

Managing the carbohydrates intake per meal is helpful in managing blood sugar elevations. Determine a healthy and sufficient number of grams of carbohydrate to eat per meal. Once you have a figure, ensure the meal does not exceed the designated amount of carbohydrates.

The Plate Method

The plate method is the most practical and easiest method of implementing diabetes fighting meal plans. You do not need to use any special tools or counting index to get it done. This method is purely about the portions size that you serve on your plate, with the emphasis on having more high fibre foods and non-starch vegetables on your plate.

It works by you dividing the plate into two halves, then dividing one half further into two, to leave you with three sections. You can even find sectionalised plates at your local supermarket. On the largest section of your plate, serve non-starch vegetables like spinach, lettuce, cabbage, carrots, tomatoes, broccoli, etc. In one of the two remaining small sections, serve starchy foods like whole grain bread, pasta, beans, green peas, chips/crisps etc. and in the remaining small section add a meat (or its substitute) such as lean beef, chicken (skinless), fish, eggs, cheese (low fat), and tofu.

To the main meal, add a glass of yogurt or low fat milk, and some fruit and you will have a healthy diabetes fighting meal plan.

Glycemic index (GI)

GI is a tool for measuring the rate by which carbohydrates elevate blood sugar levels. High GI readings mean a high level of sugar release in the blood after the food is eaten. Different types of carbohydrates digest at different speeds. The healthy way is to consume foods with low-to-medium glycemic indexes.

FOODS TO AVOID OR LIMIT

Unfortunately, most of the foods that are bad for our health are all around us and 99% of the time are hard to avoid. In fact, most of us will continue eating them unless a serious health alarm is raised. You should limit these foods to occasional treats or, if you have the discipline, avoid them completely.

Processed foods are not good for you if consumed regularly. They are less healthy than unprocessed foods and will only make your condition worse and can trigger other complications.

Stay away from or limit to a bare minimum any foods with refined sugar (white), refined flour (white) and stick to whole grains. Reduce or stop your consumption of sweets. Packed food and condiments like mustard or ketchup are not good for you either.

You are already aware of the risks soft drinks pose to your health and the limitations they put on your fight against diabetes. To the list of drinks, add alcohol which is another source of unwanted sugars. Beers and wines have a high concentration of carbohydrates and calories which are not good for a diabetic.

Chapter 5

TRUTHS AND MYTHS ABOUT DIABETIES

It's a fact - diabetes kills more people than cancer or AIDs. As much as diabetes is preventable and manageable, there are a lot of people who have no knowledge of the disease or have skewed information that could land them in trouble. Misinformation creates confusion and leads to more people unnecessarily getting the disease. Diabetes can lead to death when the right treatment or management is not applied or ignored.

Like anything that people are not well informed about, there will be truths, lies, and misinformation. Diabetes is no different. This chapter will separate the truth from the lies so that you are competently equipped with the right information to combat diabetes.

Excess weight or obesity leads to diabetes. Many people lay too much stress on obesity forgetting that there are other triggers for the development of diabetes, and that you could be overweight but your diabetes is caused by something else. Granted, obesity is a high-risk factor but will not necessarily lead to the onset of diabetes. Look out for other triggers like ethnicity, age, family history, diet, etc. After all, many overweight people do not develop diabetes.

Eat too much sugar and you develop diabetes. This is probably the most common myth of them all. Well, it is not quite true. Type 1 diabetes is mainly caused by genetics while Type 2 is primarily a lifestyle issue as well as genetics. Sugary carbonated sodas have been linked to aggravation of diabetes by spiking blood sugar levels; however, sugar is not quite the cause.

Diabetes means a special diet of bland meals; the diet for diabetics is the same diet that should be consumed by all of us; a healthy and well balanced diet. The meals of a diabetic should be healthy, just like for the one who does not have the disease and the food should just be as tasty.

Diabetes means cutting off starch. Not true. Instead, what diabetes means is cutting down on food portions and eating healthy carbohydrates. It means eating whole grains and avoiding refined flour and processed food which are high on unwanted fats and carbohydrates - which are not healthy for anyone anyway, diabetic or not.

You cannot eat chocolate or sweets. Much like the myth that you should not eat sugar because it causes diabetes, eating chocolate or sweets cannot cause diabetes or make it worse if eaten in moderation and as part of a healthy meal plan. Sweets should be eaten moderately by all.

Diabetes is contagious. Diabetes cannot be passed from one person to another directly. It is not like the common cold where if someone sneezes they can pass the germs to another person.

Diabetics are more susceptible to opportunistic illness like the cold; you are no more likely to contract diabetes than the person who does not have it. The only difference is that in those who are diabetic, it can cause more complications.

Diabetes is not serious. Diabetes is quite serious and deadly if not managed well. Diabetes has never been mild and never will be. Take it seriously. Treat and manage the symptoms with the seriousness they deserve.

Fruit is good, therefore eat as much as you can. As much as fruit is healthy and recommended, they contain carbohydrate properties which are broken down to sugar by the body. For this reason, just like other food you eat, fruits should be tracked and eaten as part of a balanced meal plan - frequency of eating, quantity eaten and the type of fruit should be deliberately controlled.

Summary

Many people have no idea they have diabetes with Type 2 hardly ever showing any symptoms. It is reported that one in every three people are unaware they have the disease. The surprising statistics about diabetes do not end there; it is also the leading cause of blindness in adults!

It is very important that you know the truth about diabetes otherwise you may unknowingly propagate the myths, lose your guard against the disease, or even pass along the wrong information. The wrong information can lead to people ignoring obvious signs about the onset of diabetes or complications thereof.

The most important thing to note about this disease is that it should not confine you or condemn you to a life that is not 'normal'. You should lead a normal, active and successful life while managing and curing diabetes. Eat like everyone else, just stick to a healthy meal plan, exercise often, and take good care of yourself.

Chapter 6

TIPS TO EFFECTIVELY MANAGE DIABETES

DRIVE OUT STRESS

The stress of dealing with diabetes is one of the biggest factors for the management of diabetes, especially Type 2 diabetes'; therefore, you need to find a way of making the situation easier on you.

Set clear goals for diabetes management have a clear and definite plan for fighting diabetes; do this and half your problems will be solved. Set meal reminders to help you have your meals on time and do not miss your doctor's appointments.

Exercise and sleep are also great for relaxing and relieving stress; physical activity will work your body and mind while sleep will give you the necessary rest to rejuvenate your body.

DAILY MONITOR YOUR BLOOD-GLUCOSE

This is a very important aspect to the management of diabetes; without the knowledge of where your blood sugar levels are, you will not be able to effectively fight diabetes. To keep things under control, take your glucose readings daily to be able to track your progress; sugar levels in the blood could be affected by many things thus the need for close tracking.

MAINTIAN PROPER FOOTCARE

As mentioned in previous chapters, one of the weakest points for diabetes patients is the foot and foot problems. Neuropathy in the foot is very prevalent in diabetics, thus the need for proper foot care.

Keep your feet clean and dry, wash in warm water and dry using a clean soft cloth or towel. Take good care of sores and injuries to the feet to avoid infection and deformities that could lead to amputation of the limb. Always wear shoes and avoid walking barefoot.

TREAT DAYTIME SLEEP AND APNEA

When you experience persistent sleepiness during the day it is likely you have sleep apnea. People that have diabetes are more likely to develop sleep apnea, which increases the risk of insulin resistance and can get in the way of diabetes management.

MAINTAIN PROPER DENTAL CARE

The risk of tooth decay and infections is quite high when you have diabetes as the excess blood sugar is also in the saliva. You need to brush and floss your teeth well, at least three times a day to eliminate the risk of periodontal problems.

MODERATE YOUR ALCOHOL INTAKE

Moderate alcohol intake is recommended for the management of diabetes; having less than two drinks per day can reduce the risk of Type 2 diabetes by around 30% in those who do not have the disease yet. As for those who are already diabetic, take very little as the carbs in alcohol can spike glucose levels in the blood if too much is consumed.

QUIT SMOKING

Nicotine is a high-risk factor for the development of diabetes. Smoking increases the chances of developing diabetes and, if you are diabetic, triggers and leads to a lot of complications. Smoking elevates blood sugar, leads to narrowing of blood vessels and heightens the risk of kidney ailments.

EXERCISE

Physical activity burns body fat and helps with weight loss. Exercise improves blood sugar regulation and response to insulin. Exercise for at least 30 minutes to an hour daily for optimal results. Engage in an activity that you enjoy and that you will remain interested in for a long time. If getting motivated or remaining consistent is hard for you, find a buddy or someone that can help you.

Conclusion

In Chapter 1, you learned what diabetes is and the several types of diabetes that are known. Despite the other forms of diabetes, the main types most of us will grapple with are Type 1 and 2, which are the most prevalent types. The pharmaceutical methods of managing diabetes is immense, costly, and seldom returns you to a 'normal' life. Once diabetes gets too advanced and triggers the onset of other problems, it can confine you to a life of suffering and unending hospital trips if not well managed.

For those suffering from diabetes, the good news is that diabetes is manageable and the complications attributed to it curable. With the right advice, attitude, and action you can beat diabetes.

You now know the right foods to eat and the proper diet needed along with the importance of exercise to effectively manage diabetes. Get on a sustained regime to boost your fitness and health. Start now and diabetes will be history before you know it.

I wish you a healthy future.

OTHER BOOKS BY INSPIRED WORD PUBLISHERS

Titles and books by our authors available on Amazon.

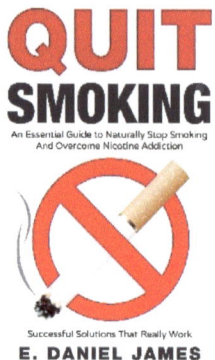

ONE LAST THING

If you enjoyed this book or found it useful I would be grateful if you would post a short review on Amazon. Your support really does make a difference and inspires others to take action and also learn how this book has helped you.

Thank you again for your support.